The Joint Pain Workout Plan

The Best Exercises for Joint and Muscle Pain Relief

By Nicholas Oetken

Table of Contents

Introduction

There are so many benefits to physical activity that regular exercise simply cannot be ignored any way you look at it.

One of the benefits of working out is that it can help to get rid of extra weight gain and to maintain your new weight once it has been lost. This is because physical activity enables faster burning of calories. Plain and simple, the more intense the physical activity is, the more calories can be burned. Increasing physical tasks such as parking farther down the parking lot at the grocery store to create greater walking distance or giving yourself more chores at home can cause you to burn more calories. But if you're really serious about burning calories, then thirty minutes of daily exercise is going to go a much longer way.

Exercise is also one of the best defenses that you have against diseases. Physical activity boosts good cholesterol levels and prevents higher levels of blood pressure, giving you a lower chance of developing heart disease. Many people who would have been patients of diabetes, cancer, stroke, and depression have been able to avert becoming so thanks to the time, effort, and investment they put into regular exercise.

If you've been feeling more tired lately and frustrated over having to do simple tasks such as picking up groceries or taking extra responsibility at work, exercise can help to boost your strength and energy by giving your body the critical nutrients it needs to aid your cardiovascular system. A healthy heart and lungs alone can give you so much more energy than you could ever ask for.

The benefits of exercise are just as much emotional as they are physical. Have you felt stressed out from all of the negative aspects of life that have taken their toll on you? Energy can stimulate chemicals in your brain that make you feel happier and more relaxed at the same time. Your confidence will be boosted significantly with the addition of exercise to your daily schedule. All the same, exercise can help you to get more sleep at night (provided that you don't exercise right before bedtime).

There are many more specific benefits of regular exercise and working out that we could explore, but space does not permit us to go any further in this book. If you are suffering from arthritis or any other kind of joint pain, than getting plenty of exercise will be even more critical. Nonetheless, you still need to know how much exercise is needed in this scenario. Too little exercise won't do nearly enough to stop the arthritis from progressing any further, and simultaneously, too much exercise can only increase the pain and result in injury. This book was written to inform you of how exercising can help joint pain, the most effective workouts for joint pain, how you can manage your muscles while suffering from joint pain, and tips for easing pain during more intense workouts.

Turn the page and read on…

Chapter One: Getting Started

If you've been suffering from joint pain or arthritis for some time now, then you've had those experiences where you want to do absolutely nothing but lay around all day. As pleasing as this may sound, it's really only bound to make your problems worse. Throughout human history, doctors and medical professionals have long been prescribing a number of 'cures' and treatments for joint pain in general, but nothing is going to help you as quickly nor as strongly as adding a strict workout regimen to your daily schedule. Those who manage to stay flexible by exercising will be able to handle their pain significantly better than the people who do not.

Working out will increase your threshold for pain. When you suffer from chronic pain, the amount of time it takes for pain to make you feel uncomfortable will be very, very short. Exercise strengthens your joints and muscles, and also makes them more flexible, in order to boost that threshold for pain.

HOW MUCH EXERCISE IS GOOD FOR JOINT PAIN

First and foremost, you should always follow the recommendations from your doctor, and you should be working out at least once every day. You want to get exercise, but you want to do it intelligently. Too little exercise (as in five minutes of running or weight lifting) is better than nothing, but it's not going to give you the benefits you desire. At the same time, over exerting yourself at two hours of work out sessions a day is only going to cause your joints to become more inflamed since you're not letting them rest.

As a general rule of thumb, thirty minutes of low intensity exercises per day is what you're going to want to shoot for. Examples of low intensity exercises include exercises on an elliptical machine, swimming, cycling, walking, etc. Many people, for the sake of convenience, will split this exercise time into two fifteen minute segments, one in the morning and one in the evening.

There are a multitude of studies that show moderate exercise to be immensely beneficial for joint pain. But again, heeding the advice of your doctor is critical, since the circumstances of your situation are going to differ from others, regardless of whether it's slightly or significantly. Coming up with an exercise plan under the guidance of a medical professional is always a good idea.

Any good doctor is never going to recommend the same workout regimen for every one of their patients. Like we have said, every patient is different, and even if one workout regimen works very well for eighty percent or more of joint pain or arthritis patients, that doesn't at all mean that it's going to work well for the remaining twenty or less percent. The point is that you should feel encouraged seeking the assistance of a professional as they know from experience what to subscribe for you.

WHAT TO DO BEFORE WORKING OUT

There are steps that you should take before each work out session. You may think that we're referring to warm ups and stretches, and that's definitely true and we'll get to it in a moment. But the first step you need to take before warming up is to understand the correct posture of the exercise. This is where seeking the help of a professional really comes into play, since many people with little to no knowledge of exercising will often put themselves at risk by adopting improper posturing while lifting weights, running, etc. For people who are suffering from joint pain, this is especially critical to watch out for.

Like we have just mentioned, stretching is also vitally important. Stretching before a workout warms up your muscles and increases the circulation of blood, allowing for more flexibility and alleviation of joint pain during the work out. There are a number of different stretches that you can use before working out, including:

- Lie flat on your back on a soft surface, with your legs raised and supported on a piece of furniture, such as a couch or chair.

- The yoga 'Happy Baby' pose, where you lie on your back and hold your knees directly to your chest.

- The Runner's Stretch, where you step with one foot forward into a lunge and then reach out to try and touch your toes with your fingers. Exhale as you straighten your extended leg.

- The Standing Side Stretch, where you hold your feet close together and then extend your arms above your head until they touch. Breathe as you slowly bend your body to the left and then to the right.

WORKOUTS THAT SHOULD BE AVOIDED

Now that you hopefully understand the importance of correct posturing and stretching before working out, let's cover one more important topic before we get into the actual workouts: the workouts that you should avoid.

Typically, people who suffer from joint problems will need to avoid exercises that are high impact. Examples of high impact exercises include running or sports like basketball. Basically, any exercise that inflicts wear and tear on the joints is a high impact exercise.

Does this mean that you should turn to a less intense exercise such as golf? Not necessarily. Sports such as tennis or golf can be problematic for joint pain because you are only rotating your body in one way. Granted, tennis is the better of the sports in this regard since there's slightly more motion, but you are still likely to use one side of your body more than the other.

By all means, if you enjoy the sports of basketball, golf, tennis, or running, then don't give up on them. They just shouldn't be your primary workout regimen if you plan on using exercise to lessen the joint pain. Both sides of your body need to be exercised. One example of a workout that we will examine is Pilates, as it involves much twisting and rotating and ensures that your entire body is involved in the workout.

If you've been suffering from chronic joint pain, or any kind of chronic pain for that matter, then you've likely experienced what a reduced quality of life feels like. But working out is one of the most effective things you can do to improve your quality of life and end those days where you can't do anything but painfully sit around the house.

Chapter Two: Effective Workouts for Treating Joint Pain

One of the best types of workouts for treating joint pain is going to be cardiovascular exercise. Numerous studies have shown a definitive link between more cardiovascular exercise and less back and knee pain.

Strength training is another exercise that has been shown to ease back and joint pain. Some people prefer to use traditional free weights for strength training, while others rely on machines that simulate support your body doesn't have. Other people prefer to use a combination of the two, or start with machines before transitioning to free weights.

Pilates and yoga are other forms of workouts that should not be overlooked. Both have been repeatedly shown to be effective at joint pain reduction, but especially in the case of someone who is suffering from chronic pain, they should first be done under the supervision of a professional.

In this chapter, we're going to examine several different workouts that have been shown to help joint pain for numerous individuals in the same position as you in the past and present. Just because one workout lowers your pain doesn't mean it will for your friend who is going through the same health problems you are; which is why we've included such a large variety of workouts in this chapter. By no means should you be performing all of these or attempting to try all of these exercises. Instead, work with your doctor to narrow down this list to a select few, and then try your hand at those.

Eventually, you should find a workout plan that keeps your joint pain down.

Without any further ado, here is the list of workouts that you can use to heal the pain in your joints:

CHAIR STAND

For the chair stand workout, sit in a normal chair, stand up, and then sit down again. All right, so this sounds like something you do every day when you sit down to work or eat, right? Not quite. The difference is that when you sit down to work or eat you just plop down without a second thought given to it. With the chair stand workout, you control how you sit down. You use your arms to assist you, and sit down slowly and carefully. This may sound like a simple exercise, but performing fifteen repetitions at a time will give you more of an exercise than you first expected.

WATER WORKOUT

This workout is especially effective for those who have joint pain. Step into a shallow pool that is no more than four feet deep, and then walk between the two ends of the pool at a brisk pace. The water's buoyancy is what will relieve the pressure on your joints, especially in your ankles, knees, and hips.

YOGA

Yoga has been widely used to treat inflamed joints, and with good reason. Nearly every joint pain patient who has tried yoga has seen positive results. The relaxation techniques in yoga will boost your immune system and reduce inflammation in the joints. Some forms of yoga will need to be avoided, such as power yoga, since they can put too much pressure on the joints. But gentle stretching is excellent for maintaining if not enhancing mobility.

While some workouts you should be able to try safely on your own at home, provided that you research them thoroughly to make sure you have the best posturing, yoga is one that would be best done with the aid of a certified professional. Consider signing up for a class that can be easily incorporated into your daily schedule.

STRETCHING

Most people associate stretching with pre-workout warm ups, and it definitely fulfills this role well. But quite a few joint pain patients like to include slightly more intense stretching as the main part of their workout. For example, place the ball of your foot through a loop, grasp the straps end with your hands, and then straighten out your leg. As you pull on the straps, lift your leg. This gives you a hamstring stretch.

Hand stretches are also excellent workouts to ease the joint pain in your fingers. Spread apart your fingers as wide as they will go, and then squeeze to make a fist. Then overextend your fingers out to their widest positions, and restart the process. This stretch is even more effective if completed under water or with a foam ball.

PILATES

Pilates is a terrific workout for arthritis patients who want to both stabilize their joints and strengthen their muscles at the same time. An example of a Pilates workout is to lie down on your back, and then bend your knees while placing your arms at each side of your body. Lift your pelvis, contract your abdominal muscles, and inhale through your nose. Exhale back through your nose as you lower your pelvis again.

WEIGHT LIFTING

Weight lifting is a good exercise for anyone, but only if you know your limits! This is definitely not an exercise where you want to over exert yourself. Weight lifting should always be initiated by performing bicep curls using light weight that weigh no more than five pounds at the most. Progressively add new weight and more sets to increase your endurance.

The primary benefit behind weight lifting is that it trains your body to lift everyday items. If you've ever felt more joint pain while hauling groceries into the car or transporting heavy boxes at work, weight lifting will accustom your joints to not flare up while lifting heavy items.

TAI CHI

Tai Chi is a low impact exercise that is a good beginner workout for someone who's just starting to use exercise to reduce joint pain. Tai Chi utilizes slow movements that are meant to enhance mobility in the body and reduce pain in the muscles and joints, making it perfect for arthritis patients. Since Tai Chi makes use of smoother movements rather than mid to high intensity exercising, slightly more time should be spent on it each day. If you would spend thirty minutes with other workouts daily, try forty minutes a day for Tai Chi.

CYCLING

Cycling will improve the joints in your feet and ankles (in addition to your quad muscles), regardless of whether you bike outdoors down a trail or with an exercising bike. Many aerobic exercises are excellent for cardiovascular health but are also high impact, making them unsuitable for many arthritis and joint pain patients. Cycling is a notable exception to this, in that it greatly benefits your cardiovascular system but is not high impact. Try cycling two or three times a week at thirty minutes each.

QI GONG

The purpose behind Qi Gong is to give you a stronger core and better posturing. Stand upright, close your eyes, relax, inhale through your nose, and exhale through your mouth. Once you've gotten this rhythm down, put your hands on your stomach to move your diaphragm with each breath you take. Strengthening your core abdominal muscles will be one of the best things you can do to give you better posturing and balance.

ELLIPTICAL TRAINING

Elliptical training is a workout that will test your endurance, but is best suited for those who are more experienced with gym training and/or are willing to sign up for a cross training class/program. Arthritis patients who desire a low-impact and high-intensity exercise will find their solution with elliptical training. Always begin with a constant ramp height and resistance, and then proceed to make adjustments in the coming weeks and months.

HIP EXERCISES

Hip exercises will aid in lowering pain in your hip joints and muscles. For one hip exercise, face your kitchen counter and hold onto something steady, such as your sink. Proceed to bring one knee up as if you were marching. Lower it back down and then repeat the process with your other knee. Complete fifteen to twenty repetitions on each knee per day. Always keep all of your toes facing forward, and extend your leg until the foot is a few inches from the ground.

Are these the only work outs that you can pursue to lower joint pain? Definitely not, but the reason why we have included these exercises is because they have been the most successful with the greatest variety of arthritis and joint pain patients. Try a combination of these work outs until you find the balance and pain relief you need.

Chapter Three: Managing Your Muscles After Working Out

Joint pain on its own is one thing, but what many people don't realize is that joint pain and muscle soreness go hand in hand. When your joints flare up, the surrounding muscles and tissue become more painful as well, and vice versa. This is why managing your muscles while working out is absolutely critical to reducing the symptoms of joint pain, especially after you've added increased intensity or time to your workouts that's causing your muscles to become sore and increase inflammation in the joints.

There's no need to get sidetracked by muscle pain or to allow it to make your joint paint worse. This chapter is about understanding the link between joint and muscle pain, and how you can maintain it properly.

THE FUNDAMENTALS OF MUSCLE PAIN IN REGARDS TO EXERCISE

It's perfectly normal if your muscles are sore after physical exercise. Sore muscles are also very likely to develop if you've done something that your body is not used to, like adding extra length or intensity to your workout, or running for many miles when you typically just take a quick jog around the block a couple of times. With that in mind, you should never be immediately alarmed if your muscles are sore after physical exercise.

Typically, muscle soreness will peak two days following the physical stress. The reason the muscles feel sore is because the added physical stress can create very small injuries within the tissue and fibers. This causes the soreness to develop in about twenty four hours, before reaching its peak at forty eight. Following the peak, it will start to get better.

Once your body has adjusted to the added intensity in exercising, your muscles will also get used to it and the level of soreness will go down over time. This is because the tissues and fibers in your muscles are strengthening and reducing the chances of them becoming injured.

That's the fundamentals of muscle pain in regards to working out and exercises. Now let's examine the fundamentals of joint pain.

THE FUNDAMENTALS OF JOINT PAIN IN REGARDS TO EXERCISE

If your joints ever feel sore, it's almost always going to be the result of inflammation, which may or may not be a sign of osteoarthritis (but usually is). The older people get, the more common inflamed joints become. This is because the cartilage that exists in the joint gradually wears away over the years, leaving the joints significantly more vulnerable to inflammation.

Granted, joint pain can also be the result of injury or physical trauma. An injury sustained to the knee can cause a ligament to be torn, which almost always leads to pain.

TREATING MUSCLE AND JOINT PAIN

If you've just added intensity or an extended period of time to your normal workout session, and bearing in mind that you're already suffering from joint pain (considering that you're reading this book) then your muscles are going to be sore for at least forty eight hours following the exercise. With each time that you continue to exercise based on the most recent revision, your body can and will adjust. But as long as your muscles are sore after each new exercise, your joints will only get worse...which will obviously only make working out more painful and result in decreased motivation to want to work out.

The best relief for a sore muscle is going to be an ice wrap, or an ice pack that is wrapped in a towel. Apply the ice to your sore muscles almost immediately in order to cut inflammation to your joints and relieve soreness simultaneously. This activity alone will almost certainly result in lessened pain for your joints. After adding ice, you can then add heat to your muscles to get the blood flowing. Heat will also relieve joint pain as more blood circulates throughout your body. At times, muscle soreness/pain is going to require more treatment than just ice and heat. If your doctor allows it, you can look into pain relievers. Some natural substances that can keep muscles soreness down include Vitamin C and other antioxidants. Protein has also been found to help keep pain down while working out.

The bottom line is that if muscle pain occurs quickly, it is a clear indication that you have been injured. But if you gradually feel more and more sore over the few days following exercise, then it's a perfectly normal sign of your body adjusting to the new workout. Nonetheless, your muscle soreness still needs to be managed in order to keep your joint pain down as well.

Remember to take your time as you ease your way into a new workout. Start light and then build yourself up over the coming weeks and months. It's nearly impossible for your joints to get nutrition without moving, and it's going to be a challenge to get moving if soreness in your muscles from yesterday's increased workout is only making your joint pain worse. That's why managing muscle soreness is quite possibly the most overlooked area of attention for those who suffer from muscle pain. Your muscles support your joints and when your muscles are strengthened; your joints are strengthened too. All the same, if your muscles are in pain or are sore, your joints are going to be in similar or worse shape.

Chapter Four: Common Exercising Mistakes with Joint Pain

Exercise helps keep excess weight down, fights back against negative health risks, and is very beneficial to your heart. But at the same time, those who fail to exercise carefully will be at greater risk for energy and joint stress. These risks are not at all strong enough to be a reason to quit exercising all together, but they are strong enough that you should exercise with caution. That means that in regard to arthritis and joint pain, you need to adopt exercising habits that will reduce your chance of sustaining injuries to your joints that will only make your problems worse and not better.

This chapter is about common exercising mistakes that people with joint pain make, and how you can avoid them.

MISTAKE #1: EXERCISING TOO MUCH

Many people have high motivation when getting ready to commit to a workout program, and while that's absolutely a good thing, it can also lead to a potential disadvantage. This disadvantage is that high motivation can encourage you to exercise too much. Once you've been exercising for over a half hour, what's to stop you from exercising for over two hours if you feel up to it? It cannot be stressed repeatedly enough that too little and too much workout will be detrimental to your joints. You need to find the right balance between the two.

If you decide to work out for two hours a day, it won't be long before your knees flare up and your entire routine comes crashing down, and in a heartbeat, you may suddenly lose all of the motivation that you just had. The reason for this is because your body needs to adapt to any routine that you give it, and your body can only adapt if you allow it to adjust over time. Fifteen to thirty minutes of workout sessions a day will be plenty. Any less or more than that will cause adverse effects rather than positive ones.

MISTAKE #2: WEARING THE WRONG SHOES

There are tons of different options for footwear that you can find for working out. Many people will purchase the lower end shoes simply to save on money, but in reality, saving money on footwear could equal increasing your chances of injuring yourself. Allow the employees at the store to examine your foot and how you walk, so that they can then decide what the best shoe will be for you. We're not saying that you should avoid the lower end shoes all of the time no matter what, but we are saying that higher end and more expensive shoes will often times prove their value. You need to find athletic shoes that are comfortable, give your feet plenty of cushion, motion control, and arch support. If you suffer a foot related injury while working out, you'll likely be paying a visit to the physical therapist's office.

MISTAKE #3: WRONG TECHNIQUE

Regardless of whether you run or lift weight, it's absolutely important that you maintain proper posturing and technique in order to avoid the chances of developing foot injury. Maybe if you go for a bike ride every day, and the seat has been positioned incorrectly, you would be putting undue pressure on your knees. Or you may be lifting weights, but lifting them in an incorrect matter that puts an unnecessary and potentially even dangerous strain on your body.

The reality is that any individual who does not have professional instruction will not know how to line up each of their joints to keep them safe. Fortunately, doing so is something that anyone can easily learn if they put the effort and attention into it. If you are unsure if you are doing an exercise properly, ask a professional or conduct your research! Simultaneously, before you do any exercise, you should always invest heavily into researching it thoroughly. Many people, who begin to workout, wanting to be on the safe rather than the sorry side, will sign up for a class or head to a gym where a certified instructor will be able to explain each exercise in detail.

MISTAKE #4: FAILING TO STRETCH BEFORE WORKING OUT

It's very tempting to want to skip the stretching session simply due to time constraints. But the truth is that as little as thirty to forty-five seconds of stretching alone should be sufficient to get your muscles warmed up and blood circulating. Not stretching before working out will make you much more susceptible to injury as your muscles are still stiff. Your muscles will also be cold, which means that they cannot absorb impact near as well if they were warm. As a general rule of thumb, three to five minutes of stretching is what you should shoot for before any workout session, but if time is working against you, than at the very least shoot for thirty to forty five seconds. If you can stretch before working out, your body will be sufficiently prepared to take the extra physical stress.

Chapter Five: Additional Work-Out Tips

While getting plenty of exercise is absolutely important, it's understandable why you may lack the motivation necessary to work out. Exercise will help to give you some pain relief, but for some people, it can also cause the pain to flare up again in your joints. This chapter will provide you with additional tips to ease your joint pain while working out.

TIP #1: WARM UP

You would be shocked to learn about how many people actually skip warming up before working out, but the number is considerably high. The reality is that exercising without warming up first can actually cause your joints to feel more pain during exercise. This is because when your tendons and muscles are stiff, your joints will hurt more, especially in older people. As little as five minutes of warming up before exercise alone will get your blood flowing and loosen your muscles. The primary reason why people skip working out at all is because time may be against them. If you are squeezed in between other commitments, even as little as thirty seconds of warm up stretches will be enough to keep your pain down while working out.

TIP #2: KEEP A LOGBOOK

Begin with the smallest amount of impactful movement and then increase until you find the moment before your joints signal pain. Maybe if you exercise on a bike at a certain speed that doesn't cause pain, but then when you increase your speed to a certain point, your joints will start to flare up. All the same, you might not feel any pain while exercising even if you increase your biking speed, but then you'll feel unusually sore in your joints the next day.

Keep a logbook with you whenever you exercise to keep track of the moment where the pain starts to flare up, and for as many workouts as you do. Also keep track of any unusual joint pain or soreness that you feel the following day. This is referred to as your breaking point or the point in your workouts where you're overdoing it.

There's no denying that exercise is great for your body, including for those with joint pain. But if you overdo exercising, the pain and inflammation can be made worse. Keeping a logbook with you is the only surefire way to know what your breaking point is for each exercise.

TIP #3: SWITCH BETWEEN EXERCISES

Most workout professionals recommend alternating between high intensity exercises and low intensity ones, and simultaneously, between working out your large muscles and your smaller ones. For example, you can alternate between exercising your legs, your back, and your arms. This will prevent you from over exercising one part of your body, and dedicating too little attention to another.

TIP #4: SHIFTING YOUR WEIGHT

Maybe you're performing lunges as part of your workout, but your knees increasingly signal to you that they are in pain. There is a way to turn this problem around. Shift your weight to another part of your body. So instead of applying weight to your knees, transfer the weight to your feet. The strain put on your knees will subsequently decrease. Or maybe you've been doing planks lately, and your wrists have become sore as a result. Instead of applying pressure to your wrists, you can instead perform the planks using your forearms.

TIP #5: MAKE USE OF PROPS

It's very easy to modify any form of work out in order to make it significantly more comfortable, and many times, the best way to modify it as such will be to make use of props. The fundamentals behind using props are very similar to the fundamentals behind why you would want to shift your weight or alternate between different exercises. For example, if the joints in your hands or wrists have been hurting from pushups, you can try holding onto dumbbells instead. This will straighten your wrists, as opposed to curving them when your hands are placed on the floor.

A more expensive alternative to simple props such as dumbbells or blocks would be high end exercising equipment, but if you don't have access to a gym or such equipment at home, then simple props like we have discussed will work well for you too.

TIP #6: STAY HYDRATED

Every workout professional will place a strong emphasis on the importance of staying hydrated while working out, and this applies even more so to people with joint pain. Being dehydrated alone can cause the inflammation and pain in your joints to get worse and coupled with the stress of physical exercise and working out, it's easy to think of the kind of pain the person may feel. Drink plenty of water not only before, during, and after working out, but throughout the day as well. Take a water bottle with you to work and then drink a small sip out of it at least once every five minutes. This alone can keep your body fully hydrated and ready for the next workout session.

Conclusion

Joint pain and arthritis can easily cause inflammation and pain throughout your muscles. Exercise may not be the absolute cure for joint pain, but it can definitely help to restore much of your lost mobility and reduce the symptoms of it. One reason why you might suffer from joint pain is because, in the case of osteoarthritis, the cartilage within your joints is deteriorating, resulting in the loss of mobility and pain that you have felt. The workout techniques that you have learned throughout this book will enable the fluid in your joints to move more freely, reducing your symptoms significantly.

However, the workout methods and strategies that you have learned throughout this book will only work for you if you fully commit to them. If you aren't sure about which of these exercises will work for you, don't be afraid to consult with a health professional. As they will tell you, regardless of which exercise method you choose to go with, you must commit to it on a daily basis in order for you to see positive results.

In fact, most medical professionals recommend that people with arthritis and/or joint pain conduct some physical activity each and every day. If you do too much exercise, you'll only suffer from more pain as your inflamed joints take on more than they can handle and can't find enough rest. But all the same, if you get too little or no exercise, the muscles surrounding your joints will become more weak, and your joints themselves will become more stiff and painful. That's why it is absolutely critical that you find not only the right workouts for you, but the right balance as well.

Once you find what works for you, you must stick with it and never give up on it.

The benefits that you will receive from the workout methods in this book will be immensely valuable for you. You'll be able to maintain a healthy weight and lower levels of stress, be more flexible with your joints, improve your balance and posture, maintain bone density around the joints, and give your joints the nourishment they need. There is no form of medication that can give your joints the same kind of benefits.

No longer will you need to be in so much pain that you don't feel up to doing anything but laying around on the couch. No longer will you need to rely only on pain pills to keep the effects of inflammation down. As long as you don't give up on working out, working out won't give up on you.

Good luck!